David

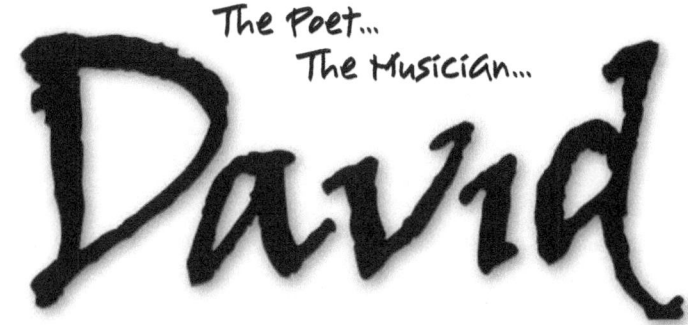

The Poet...
The Musician...

David

A Young Man's Journey Out of The Light And Into The Darkness of Bipolar Disorder

http://davidfranchini-bipolar.blogspot.com

AuthorHouse™
1663 Liberty Drive
Bloomington, IN 47403
www.authorhouse.com
Phone: 1-800-839-8640

First published by AuthorHouse 1/28/2010

ISBN: 978-1-4490-7845-4 (e)
ISBN: 978-1-4490-7844-7 (hc)
ISBN: 978-1-4490-7843-0 (sc)

Library of Congress Control Number: 2010901104

Printed in the United States of America
Bloomington, Indiana

This book is printed on acid-free paper.

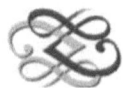

In Tribute and Honor to my Dearest Son

DAVID FRANCHINI

His Lyrics and Poems — His Battle and Rage

With Bipolar Disorder

1976 — 2008

DEDICATION

This book is dedicated to all the incredibly creative and highly sensitive men and women who struggle every moment of their daily lives with mental illness. I will always pray for them to strive for hope, courage and fortitude to never give up. There is so much beauty in our world—I wish I could enfold you in my arms and have you truly feel the power of love and admiration you all deserve.

Always yours truly,
David's Mom.... Loretta

As a mother, I write this book for my sweet son David—to honor his courage and fortitude in dealing with Bipolar; and in the last year and a half of his life with Obsessive Compulsive Disorder. (OCD)

I write this book in the hope of helping others understand the extraordinary suffering, loss of dignity, accompanied by the shame and embarrassment caused by the stigma of mental illness and painful side effects of medications.

I need to inform and shed some understanding about mental illness while at the same time tell the world some of David's story. I, his mother, honor him for all that he was. David's generosity, kindness, compassion and fortitude, had no bounds. His life had not been lived in vain; no life is. He made a difference. His journey must be told. I hope this book will accomplish that.

Countless doctors' drugs and endless blood tests, David endured so much pain; emotional and physical. He hid much from his family and friends; only through his music and lyrics did he express his sadness, rage, and loss of dignity.

Every day he would awake to the realization that without medication - (Lithium) he could experience insanity—the loss of control of brain function. How frightened he was at the needed occasional hospitalizations to adjust his medication; so often dehumanizing. I can only imagine what David felt when expressing his fear of being harmed by other patients while he slept.

Bipolar is a medical illness. It is usually thrust upon young adults in their late teens. Lithium helped David stabilize his mood, which, mainly exhibited as manic episodes. Brain scans have shown the brain is like a circuit board; the mother of circuit boards, with ideas and electrical impulses racing around the circuit.

The feeling of being on top of the world, in control, capable of doing and accomplishing several tasks and projects all at the same time— then of course... many, which do not come to fruition; consequently cause feelings of sadness, disappointment, irritability, and depression.

I wanted to write this book in order to speak up for those who cannot speak for themselves. We need officials of government to support more funding and research necessary to educate society to work toward erasing the number one problem of pain of stigma.

Hospitals and mental facilities must give better, more compassionate care to those suffering the extraordinary loneliness of battling mental illness. Our elected officials need to create legislation reducing the huge financial burden put upon the patient's family. As better funding and treatment becomes available for all young men and women who endure this pain and loss of dignity, we will begin to erase their reoccurring suffering.

The brain is an organ of the body, and mental illness is a medical illness. Individuals with mental Illness are not apart from us. They live among us as writers, artists, musicians, mathematicians, architects, poets, actors etc. They are highly sensitive, creative, and intelligent human beings worthy of love, compassion, respect, and kindness.

And to my dear son David; You are always with me in spirit. I thank you with all my heart for all the joyous times we shared; as well the sad times in which you have taught me so much. I will never forget your ironic humor and all our laughter. It is those warm and treasured memories that give me the strength and sustenance to carry on each day, as the grief at times feels almost unbearable.

Dave, we have been blessed. We experienced real love and respect for each other. I honor you each day by living my life the way I know you would want me to. Until I am reunited with you, Dad Lino, and Grandma Stella...

Ciao, il mio Tesoro (my treasure) Con Amore e Abbraccio Forte, Forte (With love & strong hugs)

Mamma

ACKNOWLEDGMENTS

I am grateful and blessed to have been surrounded by so many loving family and friends. Without their support, caring and patience it would not have been possible to undertake a project such as this, to which such emotional challenges were attached.

To my big sister Pat and her partner Kathy, my brother Steve and his wife Edna, and my dearest friend Bonnie. Thank you for always offering counsel and demonstrating your love, even when I was unbearably angry and blameful while deeply grieving the loss of my precious son David.

To Cliff and Wandalee. Cliff... From my heart to yours, I express my enormous gratitude and love to you for your guidance, assistance, and constant encouragement to me with this project. Without your collaboration, computer skills, and creativity, this task of honoring, and giving just tribute to my sweet son would be almost insurmountable.

And to Wandalee (Cliff's wife), your expressions of unconditional love and support so often pulled me out of many of my despairing moments. And as David would often write to me...

May you both experience all the best this world has to offer, along with infinite good health.

To Ivan, David called him 'Bro', for brother. To Ivan's mother and father, Consuelo, (my dearest adopted sister) and her husband Arnaldo. Thank you for always being there for David, exhibiting the utmost respect, unending love, kindness and humor. You sustained me in the most agonizing time of my life. I embrace you with my heartfelt love and gratitude.

To my dearest and treasured friend Deanna. Only during the month spent with you did I begin to feel a glimmer of healing. Gradually, the vicious anger that I had been expressing abated. Your extremely sensitive and caring nature gave me strength when I had none. Thank you for the many tears we shared and the lovely books we read to each other. I felt such peace and comfort in your presence.

To Simone, Silvio, and children. For I was enfolded in their loving, generous and compassionate arms while living with them for three months in Cattolica, Italy.

To Fioretta and Mario Prioli for their unending display of warmth and hospitality. And, for the delicious and unforgettable "Romagnoli" meals at their Hotel Marconi.

To Aldo.... Who simply understood that I needed to experience again the gorgeous countryside of Italy. The abundance of natural beauty just amazed me and lightened my heavy heart. "Grazie" for your kindness, humor, and affection.

To Evelyn Miller, Joanne Neagus, and all at the National Alliance on Mental Health Support Group. I thank them for their expression of unending compassion, advice and support all through the years of David's plight.

To Gustavo Benejam for his sincerity, kindness and knowledgeable guidance throughout my grieving process.

'Grazie Mille' (a thousand thanks) to all. Yes, my heart is bursting with gratitude and love for all of you. May you experience abundant blessings, good health, many joyous moments, and true peace.

Sempre Con Amore - Always with love

David and Loretta

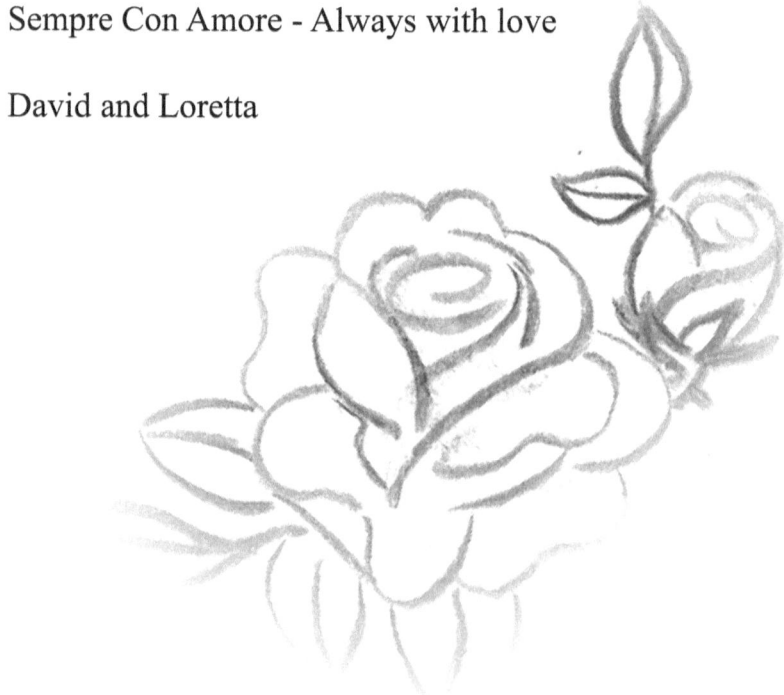

Table of Contents

DAVID

Part 1

THE YOUNG YEARS

June, 1969 I, Loretta Belarski married Pasqualino Franchini. We were so much in love and we had a wonderful dream to go back to Lino's home; a beautiful seaside village in Italy called Cattolica. We planned, worked and saved for our future and our dream.

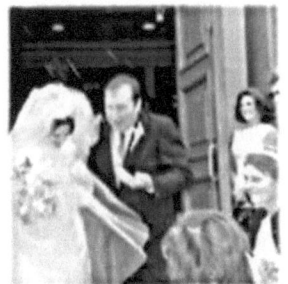 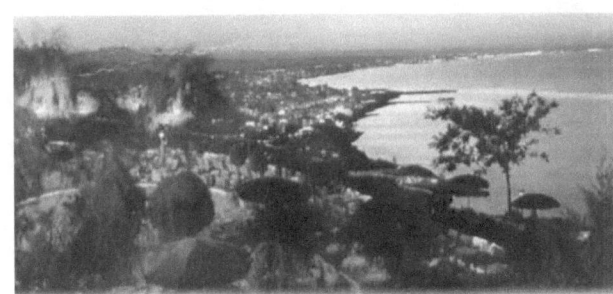

Dreams Do Come True

In 1972 it became a reality; we moved there permanently. My greatest joy occurred in 1976 when I gave birth to a beautiful, healthy boy. We called him 'David'. While Lino and I managed our small family hotel, young David was off to nursery school.

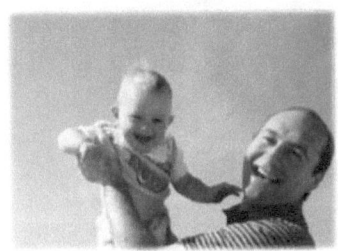 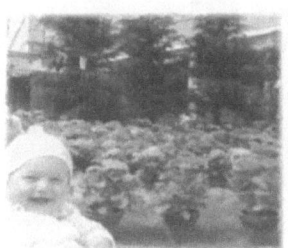 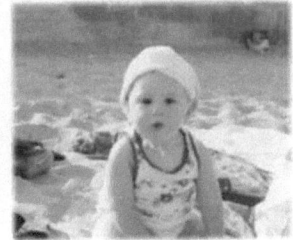

The next five years were of extraordinary happiness. The bumps on my arm come to life every time I envision "Babbo" (Papa) Lino holding David's hand as he walked him to esilo. (Nursery school) When the school day was over, David would fly out the door, arms extended into airplane wings landing in the arms of dad or myself.

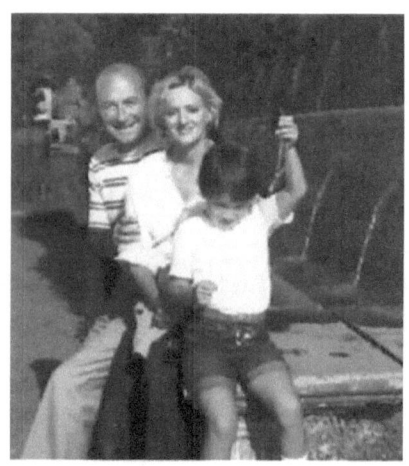

"Oh, for boyhood's painless play,
sleep that wakes in laughing day,
health that mocks the doctor's rules,
knowledge never learned in schools."
—John Greenleaf Whittier

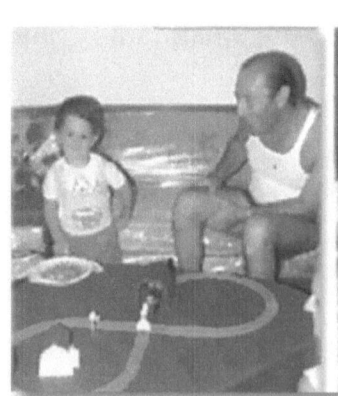 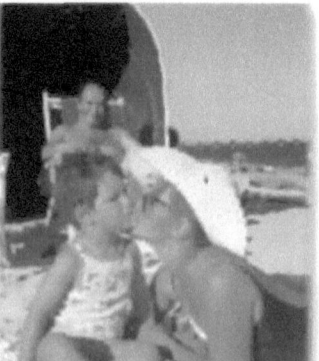 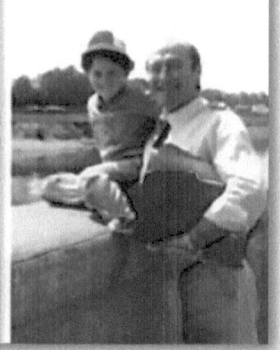

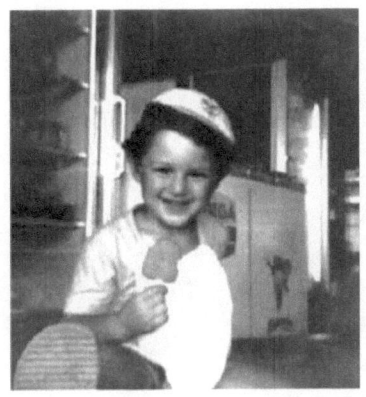

What fun for David when Grandma Stella would take him for summer walks and eating ice cream at Pimpi's Caffé.

There were so many good times. The trips to the mountains for sledding and skiing—the visits to Sicily to climb hills, pick flowers and go to the beach, even with David's occasional bouts with Bronchitis.

Truly, this felt like heaven as we all attended the lovely and quaint hilltop Castel di Mezzo Church. As the sun filtered in, it created a warm, sunlit environment.

'La Guitarra'

David was given his first guitar on his eighth birthday and shortly after he began his music lessons. He had a great feel for music; always dancing to the rhythms as soon as he could walk. Dave was our 'little performer', always singing and strumming his guitar for our enjoyment.

I was thrilled that he was musically inclined like his father Lino. David's way of being was 'allegro' (Joyful), 'happy-go-lucky'! Both my husband and I felt so thankful and fortunate for David's gay disposition.

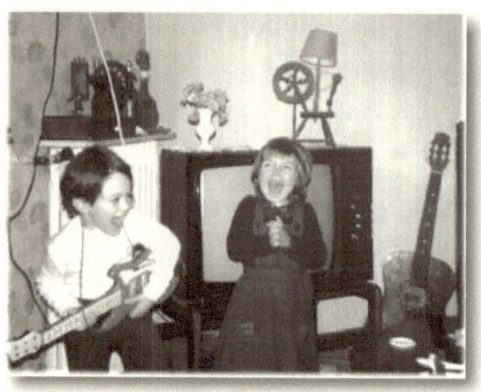

The Guitar
A New Passion

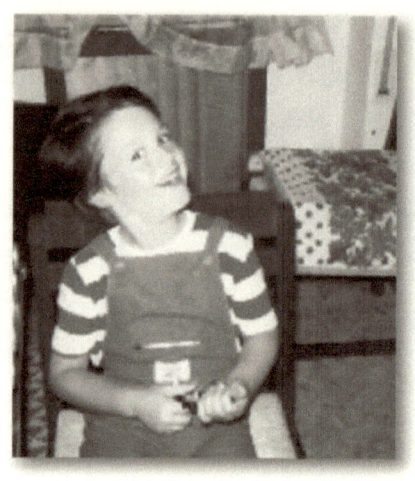

"Allegro" (Joyful)
"Happy-go-Lucky"

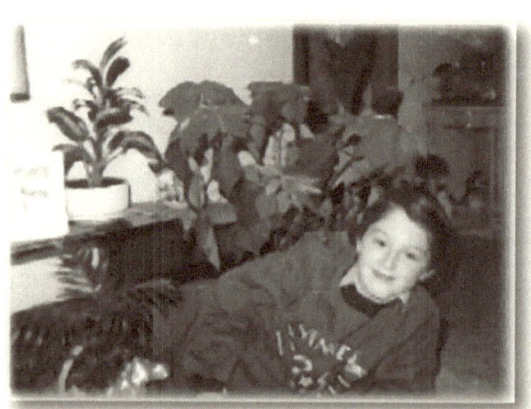

I felt incredibly grateful for so many blessings—a wonderful husband; a man of integrity, compassion and joy, and a beautiful, healthy, fun loving son.

I was living in Italy—the "garden of Europe" amid beauty and art. To add to my abundant fortune, I had the gift of many friends—true friends who always honored their word. Today, thirty years later, I cherish and honor them. Many of my friends children were of the same age or close to Dave's, and together we celebrated the yearly holidays and events.

The Italian "Carnivale" in February was one that David particularly enjoyed. All children dress in elaborate costumes and celebrate at parties in nearby castles or at gorgeous mountain-top homes and restaurants overlooking the Adriatic Sea, and lush green vineyards!

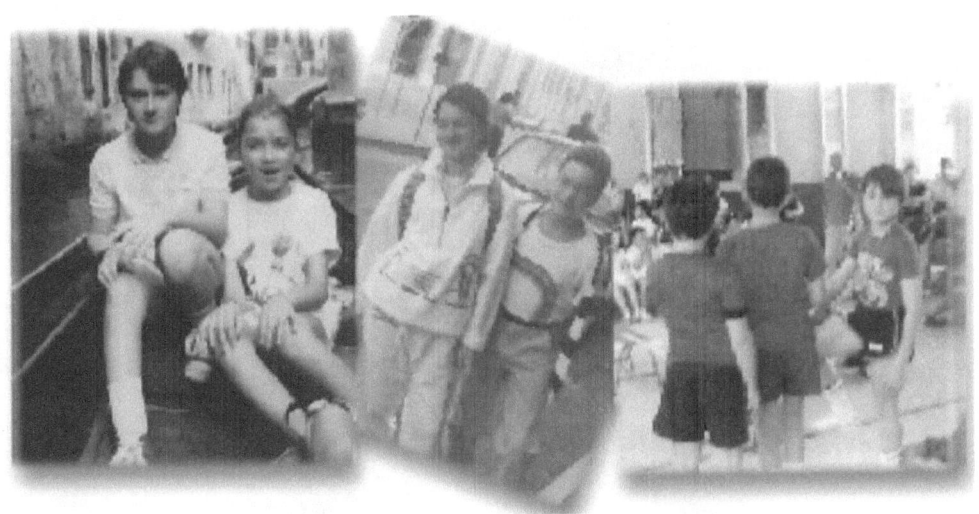

I recall two vivid memories. One is of David dressed as Luke Skywalker from the film 'Star Wars'. The other was when at twelve years old he dressed up as Michael Jackson, the famous entertainer.

David was especially close to Ivan, —he called him 'Bro', for Brother, and Lello (Rafaelle). They had so much fun creating robots from old 'stuff', playing basketball, practicing Karaté and bike riding around our little town.

They loved swimming and diving at the beach. All did fairly well in school and before long they graduated "Prima Media" - elementary school, and continued on to "Seconda Media" — middle school in the nearby town San Giovanni in Marignano.

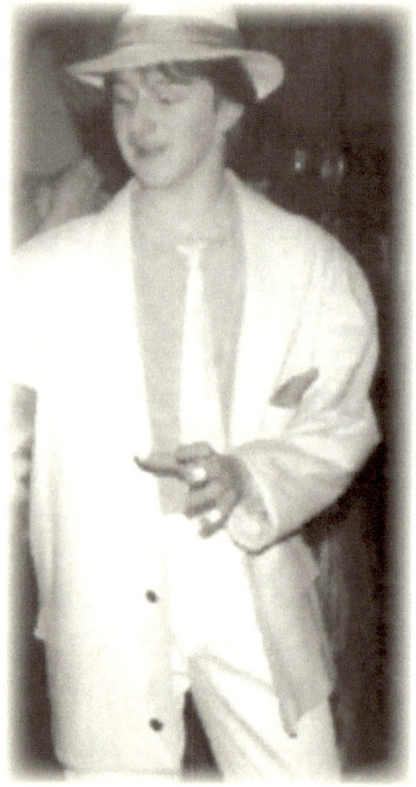

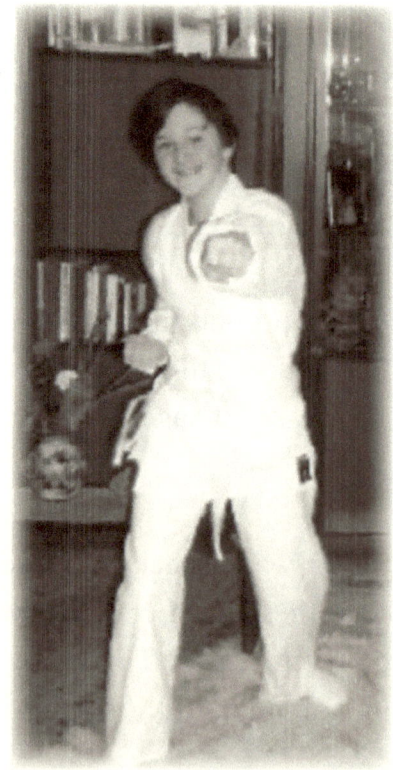

As a family we experienced some fabulous sight-seeing vacations to Venice, Rome, Sorrento, Perugia, Florence, and Sicily. We'd leave right after the closing of our little hotel, "Ideale" in September.

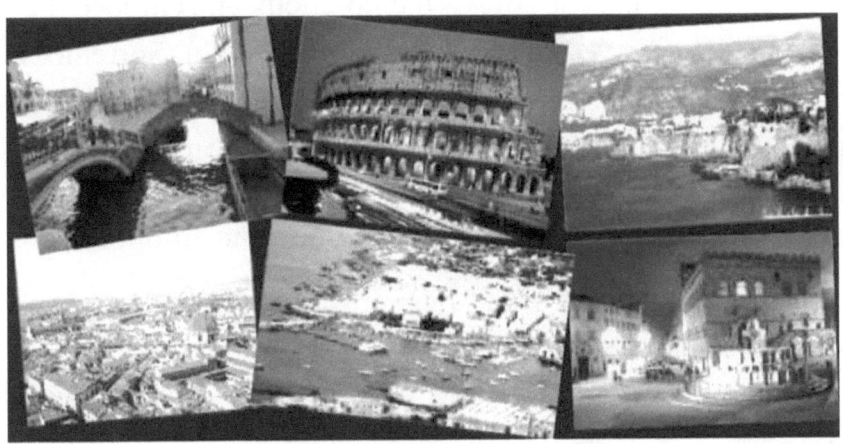

So often, I would observe Dave happily on the back of his Dad's "motorino" (motor bike) taking off to discover tiny villages in the countryside and hunt for wonder-filled treasures. They would return with adventurous stories, fresh picked flowers from a found "podere" (farm), or grapes from a vineyard.

I remember Lino climbing a tree to pick an Indian fig in Taormina, Sicily so that David and I could taste it's juicy sweetness. That was typical of his dad—passionate about life.

Many times, Lino would pick up David after his karaté lesson and they would meet me at a local "trattoria" (small family restaurant) to enjoy the typical "piadina"—(a small round crisp flat bread) with melted grilled cheese, eggplant, stuffed mushrooms, and arugula. Oh, it was so delicious.

We ran along the beaches of Agrigento, Sicily and climbed the famous ruins there. We prayed in the cathedrals of Cefalú, Sorrento, Perugia, Florence, and Venice. We stood in awe of the great works of Michelangelo—'The David', the statue of which our son was named after.

I was soon to find out that all would come to an abrupt end... Sadly.

Part 2

THE 12 to 19 YEARS
"Good Times Sad Times"

August 7, 1989. David's Dad dies of Kidney failure at fifty three years of age. David watched his father being put into an ambulance only to never return home.

Upon Lino reaching the hospital in Pesaro, Italy, his speech was becoming incoherent. By early morning he was in a coma. His kidneys and adrenal glands had stopped functioning. My sweet husband Lino passed away three days later, August seventh, 1989.

> *"Heads are down waiting for peace to come,*
> *No one sleeps now that the sun is gone."*
> —David Franchini

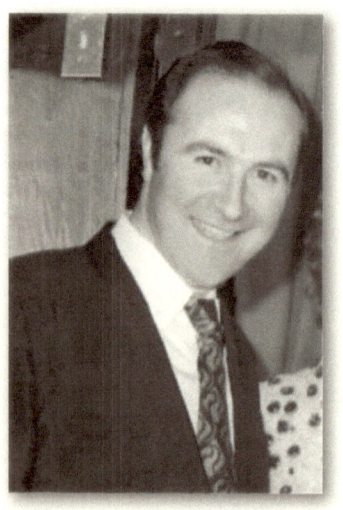 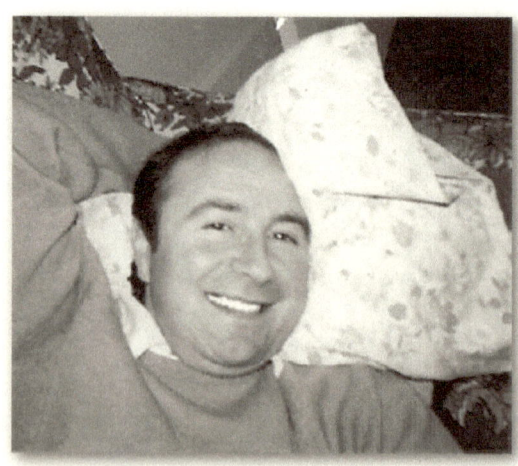

I knew in my heart David's reaction demonstrated extreme emotional pain and suffering. He took all his father's framed photographs and turned them flat down. He absolutely refused to go to bereavement counseling and never spoke about his dad.

We were both in shock—our hearts broken. A few days later, my sister Pat left California and arrived in Cattolica. She helped me with the preparation of the funeral and for our return to the United States.

Before making my final decision, I discussed it with David. He too, anxiously wanted to leave Italy. At that time, there was a celebration of American culture and fashion. Young children, especially teenagers, were attracted to popular U.S. brand name jeans and sneakers.

David had made quite a few trips to Florida where my mother and brother lived. He said he was excited and welcomed the decision. Looking back, perhaps both of us wanted to escape the pain of not having Lino with us.

'New Beginnings'

A month and a half later we were beginning a new life in Florida. Both of us had enormous loving support from my mother Stella, my sister Pat, and my brother Steve.

David started the seventh grade in September 1989. His teacher was wonderful and introduced him to another young Italian boy, Richard.

They became really good friends. Dave spent a great deal of time with 'Rich' and his family, enjoying their warm hospitality and delicious Italian meals.

After learning how to drive, I began studying at Florida Atlantic University. In 1993, I received my Bachelor's Degree in Art. Two months later, I was teaching at a nearby pre-school.

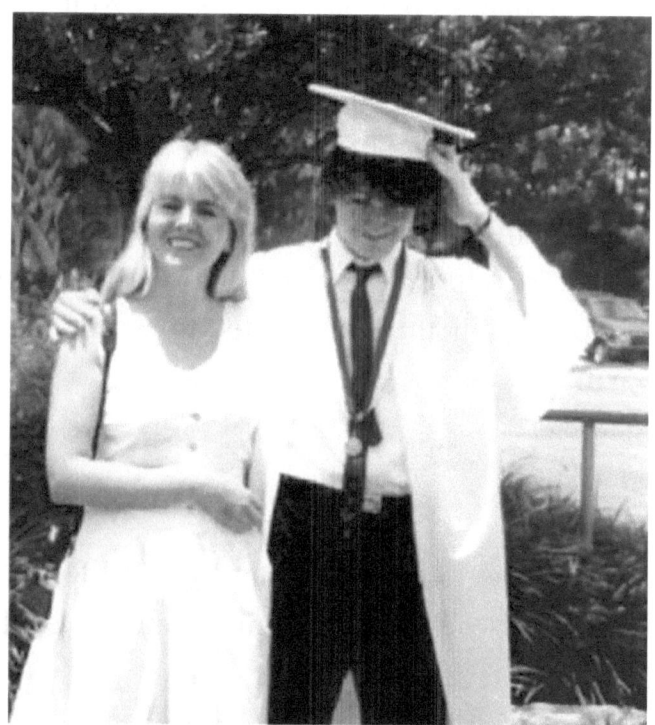

A Favorite Teacher of Dave's

'My Normal, Typical Teenage Boy.'

David was very close to my brother Steve. They built a huge skate board and ramp together. Everything seemed to progress in a positive way.

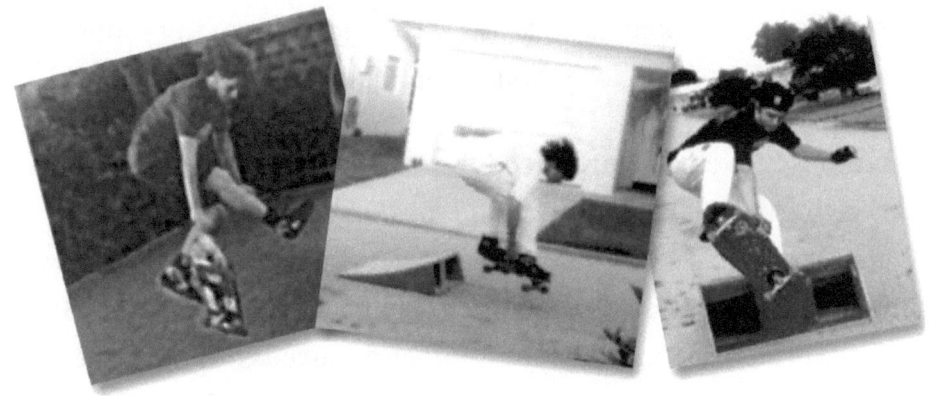

Dave And The Band - And So The Music Begins

Music was always most important to Dave. He continued his guitar lessons, singing, writing songs and lyrics, and the study of written music in a Coral Springs music school. How he loved his music. It becomes a major focus and passion for the rest of his life. He was quite industrious and worked at all kinds of odd jobs— saving money for a new guitar, speakers, microphones and distortion amplifiers.

My brother Steve had introduced him to the "Corrupted Mind" band. After trying out, Dave joined and became their lead guitarist and vocalist. At fifteen years old, he was performing "gigs" in Tampa and Gainsville, Florida. He also competed in "The Battle Of The Bands" in Coral Springs. Becoming "famous" and "successful" was the bands main endeavor. These were exciting years filled with hope for a studio contract and a tour!

"Blast to the Beat, Jump to the Tempo
Get up, Get Movin, Can You Feel It - Come on"
— David Franchini

Ahhh, the lyrics of the uncluttered mind of a typical teenager. As the years progressed I began to see a much more sophisticated style...

Yearns to Drive at 15½

David learned how to drive in his grandma Stella's 'old car'. It was a faded red. Dave called it "pink" and begged me to have it painted black— after all, what self-respecting teenage boy drives around in a pink car. So we did. David received a restricted license.

Grandma Stella loved him dearly. Often, when I was studying at the University, she would pick him up after high school dismissed and make him special snacks and dinners.

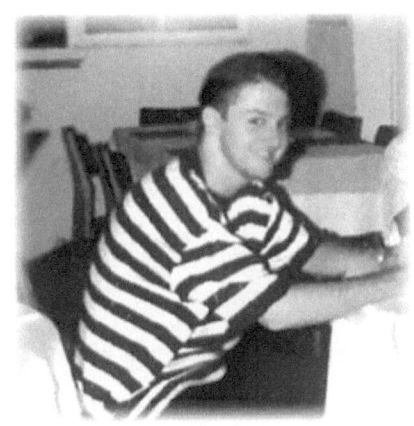

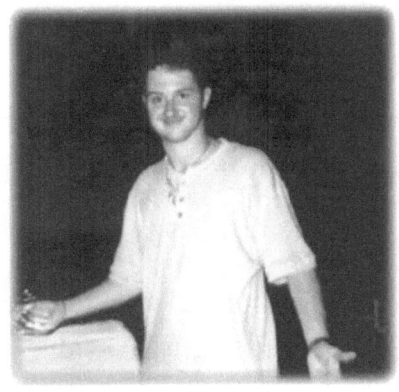

There Seems To Be a Calming Down

During this period, I felt calmer and satisfied. I believed we had come through the tragedy of his father's passing. However, it may have been too quick to pass this judgement. Perhaps it left a traumatic impression on David's brain.

As I have expressed previously, he never wanted to reveal his feelings about his Dad. I tried along with my family and friends to convince him to go for counseling, but it was always too distressing for him.

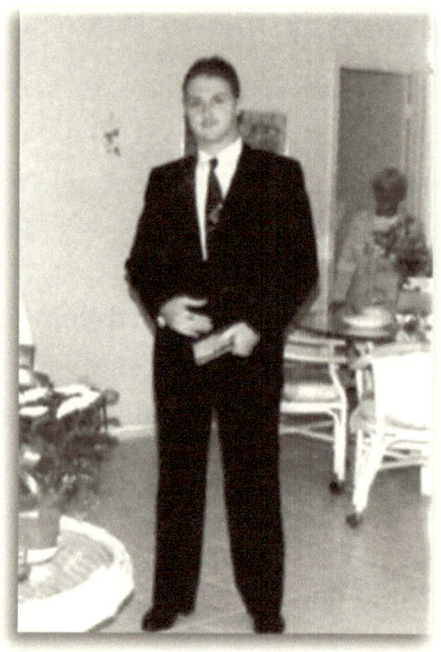

I recall that there was only one outburst of anger when he was seventeen years old. It was in June, close to graduation and his preparation for the Prom. Unexpectedly, he shouted at me, "you don't know how it feels not to have a father!" I truly had no idea what it was like for a son to experience such a profound loss of his Dad. It had been five years since Lino's passing.

Dave had graduated eighth grade and was now attending Cardinal Gibbons High School. Six months before graduation, the Dean insisted that he cut his shoulder length hair. He had complied in Junior year and literally cried for hours over it! I personally went to the Dean to ask for leniency.

I explained to him that my son was a fine, respectable, responsible young man, and that he played in a professional band. He was always accompanied by a parent when performing on the weekends. "Couldn't David simply tuck his hair up under a cap?" I asked.

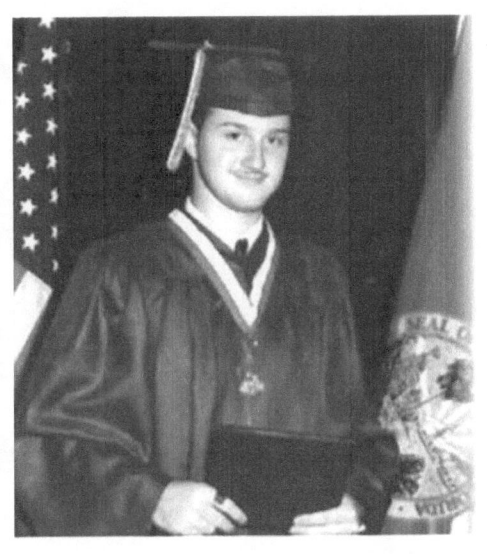

"No", was his response; "there were rules to be followed." David was dismissed from the school.

After consulting with my son, we agreed he would transfer to Coral Springs High School. Consequently, he graduated from there, on schedule, June 10, 1994.

Dave adjusted fairly well to change; he easily made new friends. Because we owned the hotel in Italy, he decided to major in Hotel Management at Palm Beach Community College.

As a young college student, he was always in need of "extra cash". He worked first at telemarketing. And then, at calculating mortgages for a local company in Boca Raton. In the evening you would find him greeting guests at the reception desk of the Boca Hotel and Resort!

He never wavered from his dream to achieve success and fame for his band. He continued playing guitar, singing and writing lyrics.

He met another young musician who helped and influenced Dave's interest in electronic keyboards and music, and their effects. They joined together to form another band called "Oblivion".

Now David was performing in two bands, studying full-time at Palm Beach Community College, and working too many hours—thank goodness for summer breaks!

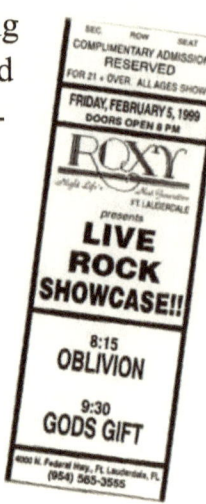

*"Pick up the pace, break out of control
Feeling the vibe dig into your soul"*
— David Franchini

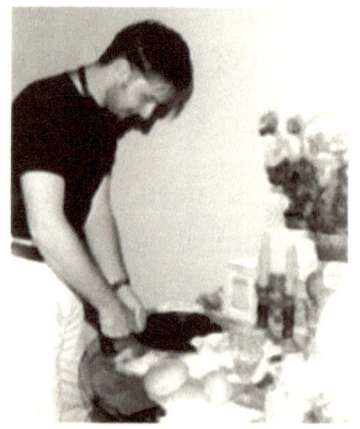

Summer Vacations in Cattolica

Dave would return to Cattolica for summer vacation and, of course, visit with his friends. David's best friend Ivan had always kept in touch. His Italian grandmother Maria showered him with her love, attention and incredibly delicious Italian cuisine!

*David's best friend
His 'Bro' Ivan*

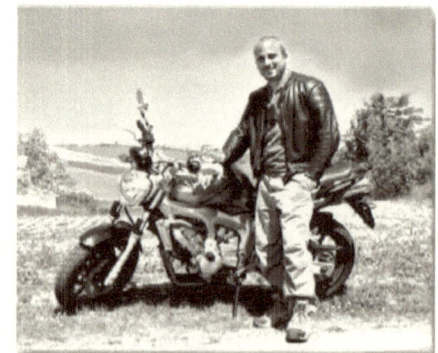

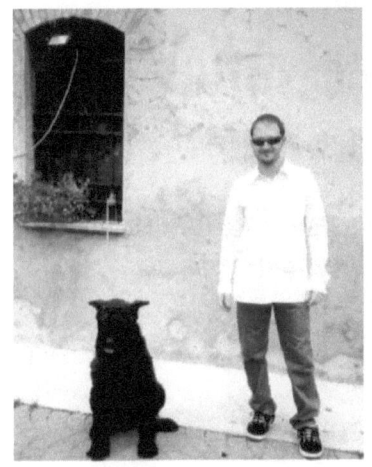 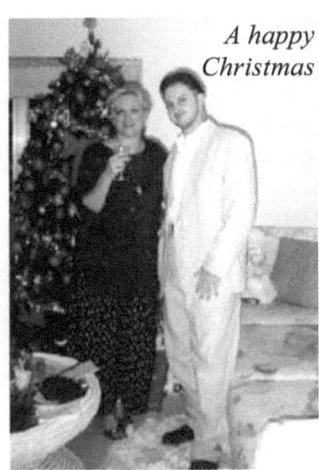

A happy Christmas

*** As of this writing, I received the wonderful news that Ivan, is engaged to be married. This joyous occasion will take place in June, 2009.

This brings many tears of joy to me—as well as some tears of sadness knowing that David would have been so proud and happy for his best friend. For he was to be Ivan's Best Man!

All my love and congratulations to Consuelo, (my dearest adopted sister) and her husband Arnaldo. As I witness the ceremony, I know I will feel David's presence as he would have not missed this moment for the world.

Change Occurs - Something's Happening

"Rearranging mental process disconnecting
Single fragment turning into deadly treatment
Tested research double-blinded system damaged"

— David Franchini

Part 3

Bipolar Disorder
"A Drastic Change Occurs"

"On your own, your plans just fall apart
You can feel the needle in your heart;
All is lost and don't know where to start"
— *David Franchini*

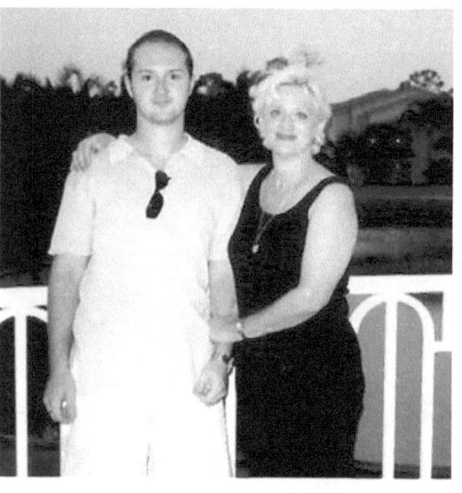

I recall vividly, September of 1998, when David returned from summer vacation, he was not the same. At nineteen he lit up a cigarette; he had never smoked.

He was very thin and had dark circles under his eyes. It was like he was detached—more secretive.

I was concerned. However, a general physical exam revealed nothing. This is when I began my "cooking frenzy" with the objective to help him gain weight.

In October, the day after Halloween, when I returned home from teaching, there, lying on David's bed were twelve plastic bags with his clothes in them. He said he was moving into an apartment with a male friend, not too far from our home. "What!", I exclaimed, you never gave me the slightest idea that you wanted to leave home. How would he manage college, work, and rent?

Was This David Growing Up? Or Signs of Something Else Happening?

Upon reflection, I thought he was trying to be independent; to be on his own and manage adult responsibilities. But in actuality, this departure certainly was not well planned, but simply impulsive behavior. Shortly, he left his friends apartment and moved in with a girlfriend. She was Italian, and both her and her mother worked in a local health food store. I felt apprehensive about it all.

> *"Breaking all the walls I see, and searching endlessly*
> *I ask the reason why, the meaning of our bleeding."*
> — *David Franchini*

David was nineteen and a half and all things began to fall apart. His friends from the band, 'Corrupted Minds' called to tell me that they were letting David go. He had stopped making rehearsals and was acting strange. He traded in his new car, (a special gift from his Italian grandmother) for an old, used corvette. Broward Community College suspended him from classes.

> *"Living through emotions left aside*
> *Digging in, damaging your pride*
> *Take away this emptiness inside"*
> — *David Franchini*

I summoned up courage, most certainly with the Lord's help, and brought him home. I began to nurse him back to a better state of physical health. Emotionally, he was somewhere else. All he wanted to do was sleep in the daytime and stay up during the night. I was desperate and determined to understand what was happening to my son.

Could He Be Using Drugs?

My family thought he was using drugs. David was disgusted and humiliated at the insult. He firmly insisted he "never did drugs". And I believed him. However, to appease my family, I convinced him to have a physical exam and a blood work-up; he complied.

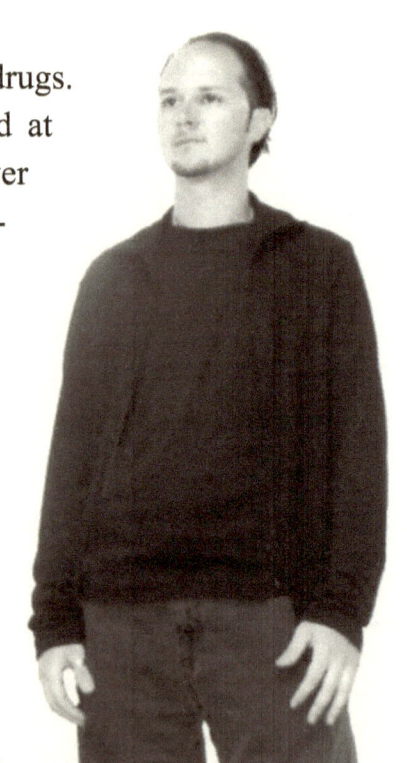

The doctor's wife indicated to me that no drugs were present. The doctor himself could not tell me because David was over eighteen years old and it was against the law to give me, the mother, information. Immediately, I knew it had to be some form of mental illness.

What Should I Do Now? A Most Excruciating Decision...

That afternoon, I made the most painful decision of my life. I went through the proceedings to "Baker Act" my son.... To legally force him to be put into a psychiatric hospital in order to diagnose his illness. A court official explained that it could take one to three days before they 'pick him up'.

That same evening, a horrifically hard knocking at my door frightened us both. David jumped up from the couch. My mother, Dave and I had just finished dinner and he was saying to me, "Ma, it's good to be home and relax".

When I opened the door and the officers came in and approached David, he looked at me terrified. "Ma! What are you doing? Ma!"

I cannot forget the expression on his face—one of incredible shock, betrayal, and at the same time while pleading, "Don't do this!" His huge brown eyes desperately expressing utter sadness and disbelief.

I felt such despair. I cried out, "I have to save you David. You'll die if you don't get help. I love you". He quietly left offering no resistance as the two officers escorted him to the police car.

I painfully watched him leave. I closed the door to my home, and with my frightened mother watching, I fell to my knees crying brokenhearted.

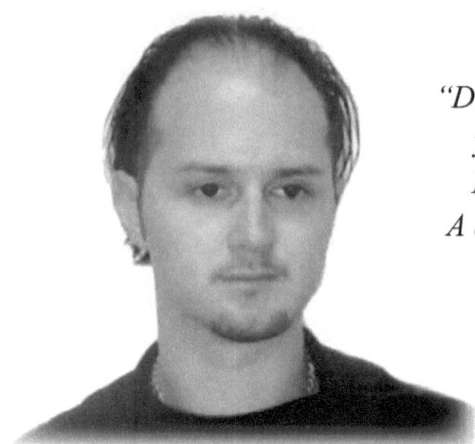

"Drowning in this life we live,
your falling in too deep.
Is there a different way?
A different way to see this?"
— David Franchini

And So The Battle Begins...

The next day, a doctor from the hospital called to inform me that David had a condition called Bipolar Disorder. He was exhibiting most of the symptoms.

Yes, 'the battle had just begun'. The search for answers to so many questions. How to help my son recover? David was prescribed Lithium and Klonopin.

The following will give some understanding about this condition affecting one's moods—known as Bipolar Disorder.

Seeking Help
David's Symptoms and Behavior

Some of the behaviors that David exhibited in the beginning of his illness were disturbing and frightening to me. He started to lose weight and not sleep at night. He had tremendous energy and would continually pace back and forth while talking rapidly. He jumped from one idea to another many times making no sense to me. I could not comprehend the meaning of what he was discussing.

David was always impeccably neat. When he stopped washing and changing his clothes, what was I to think? Things began to disappear. Where was the guitar he loved so much? Or his television? I received the phone call from a police officer at 4:00am in the morning informing me that David was confused and wandering the streets with his laptop in hand unable to find his car.

I arrived home one afternoon only to overhear David on the phone, demanding from Sony Records to draw up a million dollar contract for his band. His employer called to inform me that David was checking his car every ten minutes for fear that there was a bomb in it. He began the trading of cars, eight times in a three month period.

He had an impulsive need for things that would create a sense of excitement, self-satisfaction, and importance. There was no thought of consequences. He had no idea how very ill he was. As I previously explained, I sought medical help through the "Baker Act" where David was hospitalized and diagnosed with the condition; Bipolar Disorder. He was prescribed Lithium and Klonopin immediately. *(See page 73 for an explanation of the "Baker Act")*

The Need To Know...

I went to the library to read and learn about these various medications. A librarian tapped my shoulder and handed me two books. I devoured them desperately trying to understand all about this disorder. In the back of the one book was the telephone number of the 'National Alliance on Mental Illness'. This organization educates those dealing with mental illness in their families.

I called them immediately and the following Sunday, a course called 'Family to Family' would commence. Even though the class was full, they made an exception and said, "Yes, come and participate." I was given an exorbitant amount of information about all brain conditions and various drugs. They gave me a sense of hope that David could live a healthy and happy life, with the proper medication and adherence. I will always feel a heartfelt thanks and deep gratitude to all for their compassion and kindness.

Support groups would meet on various days of the week and I attended them for many years. It was a safe and encouraging environment whereby everyday difficulties were discussed, and solutions proposed. We dealt with issues pertaining to medical insurance, hospitalization costs, the myriad of drugs, their effects, the difficulties to adherence to medications, and problems with stigma and low self-esteem. I learned the importance of seeing my son as David, and not his condition.

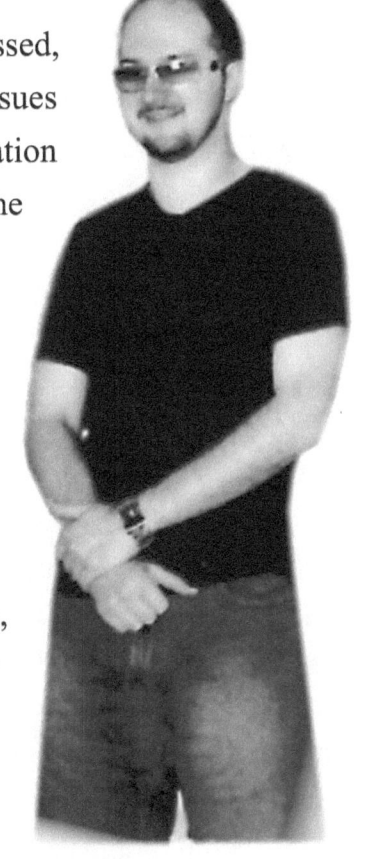

I did not want him dependent on me, his mother. My deepest desire was to foster in him a sense of responsibility, independence, and freedom of choice. Yet if he needed my help, of course, I was there for him. This was not easy by any means, but certainly worth the effort.

> *"Rearranging mental process disconnecting*
> *Single fragment turning into deadly treatment*
> *Tested research double-blinded system damaged"*
> — *David Franchini*

David suffered terribly with the diagnosis of his mental illness. In the beginning he denied it wholeheartedly. He felt so strongly the stigma attached to this condition. It took years for him to adhere to his medications. Several times hospitalization was required to adjust the doses of his "meds" until he was at a balanced level—not too low to be ineffective, or not too high to be toxic. Blood tests were done every three months.

After about five years, David realized and began to accept the fact that he could not miss taking his "vitamins" as he chose to call them. Caffeine and alcohol was absolutely avoided.

David was doing very well. After residing a few years in Italy, he negotiated the sale of our small 'Hotel Ideale' in 2004. In late November he returned to Florida settling permanently in Boca Raton. I was thrilled that he was back in the United States.

He bought a beautiful condominium and together we shopped for furniture. He decorated his home and set up a fabulous state of the art music studio. Dave was playing his guitar, keyboards, writing lyrics and working on the completion of his CD.

The whole family was so happy. David was "back" and participating in all our holidays. We enjoyed four fantastic years of good times.

It was Christmas Season of 2007 that I noticed one late afternoon, David circling his car. He was repeatedly tapping the hood, the trunk, and the gas tank cover. It took about twenty minutes to check and close his car before finally walking away. I commented, "Dave, do you know how long it took you to lock up your car? "What's happening?"

He said, "Mom, it's a new car and I have to be careful". That was true, so I dropped it. In retrospect, I should have questioned it further.

In March 23, 2007 David telephoned me, and I quote him; "Ma, I think I have O.C.D." (Obsessive Compulsive Disorder) "Please bring me some water and food... I'm all out of water and food". When I arrived, I was shocked to see him lying on the couch, his face so pale and drawn. I never saw this coming. His psychiatrist explained that O.C.D. is a co-morbid condition.

Some people will develop it if they have Bipolar. It attacked my son so aggressively that the doctor decided to treat it in the same manner—aggressively.

David would gradually go from 50mg to 300mg of Luvox (fluvoxamine). In the beginning of his treatment, lower doses weren't helping him. Therefore, Dave decided to admit himself to the hospital for fear of a manic episode occurring while taking the higher dose. That was a strong possibility.

He thought it was best to be strictly under the doctor's care. It took tremendous courage on his part to go through with this. No one wants to go into a psychiatric hospital voluntarily. It is extremely disturbing to go through the admittance procedure. Once in, one is witness to the extreme suffering of so many young men and women with severe depression and their tragic attempts at suicide.

After seven days, he returned home only to begin a harrowing therapy program. In order to alleviate the 'torture' of O.C.D., David began 'exposure and response' therapy.

He had to relearn how to do the simple tasks of everyday living. Dressing, tieing one's shoes, washing one's hands, opening a door, etc. It

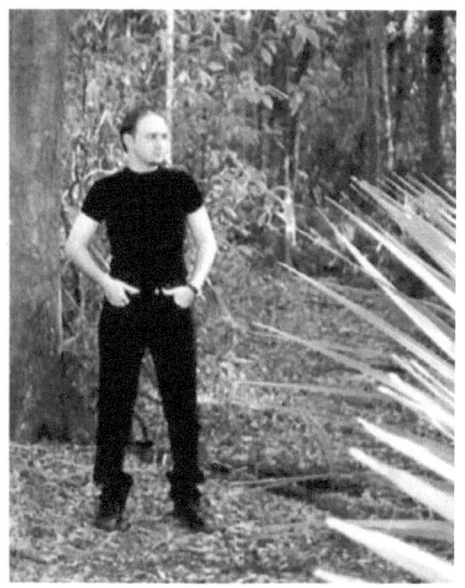

was devastating for him. It destroys ones pride and self-esteem. He fought this condition with all his strength.

Upon the completion of twenty two sessions, his therapist said, "Dave, you came through this amazingly well. You mastered the techniques and you don't need to make another appointment." It had taken seven months and we joyfully celebrated that milestone.

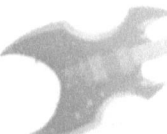

"Losing control, another broken day
Wonder aloud, I've got to get away."
— *David Franchini*

Tragically, it was not over. The medicine Luvox, created havoc in Dave's body. Severe stomach cramps, loss of his appetite, weight

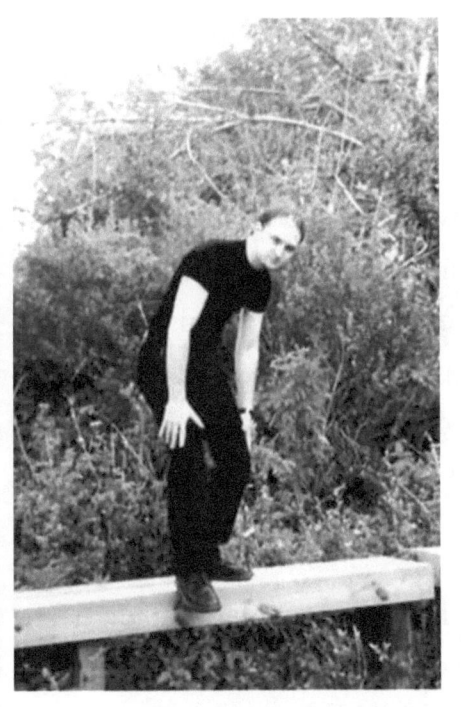

loss, and so often, dreadful diarrhea. But for my son, the worst humiliating symptom was incontinence. Already, the affects of lithium had taken a tremendous toll on his health with bouts of severe acne, hand tremors, nausea, constant thirst and hypothyroidism. (David had developed a Lithium-induced nodule on his thyroid). How does one tolerate this onslaught? As if Bipolar was not debilitating enough!

Feeling so much anger and pain, David lamented once, that he could deal with the affects of Lithium, but not with the O.C.D. medications. In his angry words, "it's f___king torture." His psychiatrist would not lower his dose either. I do believe that David feared what that could do to him. He hadn't experienced a manic episode in many years.

"Chasing obsessions until they kill;
Programmed reaction that follows your will
Exit this system that shapes your path"
David Franchini

He was just so exhausted with the never-ending doctor visits—the primary care doctor for blood tests and skin problems, the psychiatrist for his "meds", the therapist for the O.C.D. sessions, the endocrinologist for thyroid problems, and finally, the dentist for his decaying teeth caused by dry mouth form the medications.

How extremely painful for David to wake up everyday and ingest all these medications and deal with their horrendous side affects. On June 24, 2008, I met him for dinner, however, before leaving his apartment, he wanted me to listen to his latest music CD. He had just finished recording it. Enthusiastically, I expressed how much I loved it. I thought several of the songs would be great for movie sound tracks. He looked at me with his sweet, shy-like grin and humbly said, "thanks ma."

We ate at a nearby oriental restaurant; he was particularly quiet. Afterwards, we had a coffee at his favorite caffè. During our conversation, he mentioned that it was quite a while since his last girl friend, and he thought he'd join an internet dating service.

He then gave me his IPOD so that I would listen to his songs on my computer. Surprisingly, ten minutes later, he asked for it back explaining that he wanted to add two more songs. Reluctantly, I returned it to him, but I felt a sadness.

We drove back to his home. I hugged him good night saying, as always, "I love you dear, take care." From inside my car, I watched him unlock his front door without any difficulty—no repeating or checking. My heart ached for him as I sensed his deep loneliness.

"Chasing my obsession, digging in so deep
Grabbing your perfection, lay me down to sleep"
— *David Franchini*

In the following three weeks, David called several times to tell me he was doing fine. He helped me correct a computer glitch, and told me not to worry about finances. Dave always chided me about working so hard and that I should learn to "chill". (One of his favorite expressions)

"Mom, do you know how much I love you?"

Now, in the past, he could only demonstrate his love in written words, in a birthday or holiday card. Therefore, it was a real surprise, and so wonderful to hear him express his feelings so openly. I was truly touched by it. And of course, I responded, "yeah Dave, I do know; I love you too."

Dave was so generous. He showered me and my family with so many gifts. He bought us televisions, stereo systems, expensive watches, diamond rings and necklaces. On Mother's Day, David appeared at my door, arms enfolded with forty eight long stemmed red roses. He couldn't do enough, explaining that years ago, living on disability, he couldn't afford to buy us anything. Now, he wanted us to enjoy it all.

"All these actions of purity; seem so clear - yet obscure to me
As I try to understand, how you think, and where you stand
I deny - this perfect view - a perfect world we drown into."
— *David Franchini*

"Check David, Check David"

Friday, August First at 2:15am, I awoke suddenly from my sleep with the words repeating in my head; "check David, check David". I frantically searched for the keys to his apartment until five in the morning, but to no avail.

Panic—Saturday morning I drove to his place; his car was parked in front. I pounded my fists at his door and loudly called out his name over and over. There was no answer. I ran to the back of the building and kept on screaming his name.

I then recalled that he told me he wanted to make a trip to the Bahamas. Perhaps he took a cab to the airport. One time, when he was in Italy, he did go on a 'mini' vacation to Paris, France, never telling anyone that he was leaving. I calmed down, trying to think rationally. After all he was a young adult; thirty one years old. Uneasily, I departed but I couldn't relax. I was too worried about him.

The following day, Sunday August 3rd, I returned with my brother Steve. After searching the back of David's apartment, Steve had noticed that the glass of the bedroom window was shattered! It had a hole through it. I never saw that the day before. I ran to the front of the house.

Bending down on my knees, peering through a tiny opening in the kitchen window blinds, I could see that the television was on. Hysterically, I screamed out his name while banging on the window and door. My brother called the police. They arrived and proceeded to break down the door and entered the apartment wearing horrific looking gas masks.

I couldn't believe what was happening. I felt such terror, I was shaking uncontrollably. An officer asked me to go with a neighbor. In her home, she was so kind, consoling me as I sat frightfully waiting to learn what was occurring.

The Unthinkable...

David had taken his life days before with a bullet to his precious head destroying his brain. The ultimate rage, ridding himself of the part of him that he despised.

The toxicology report revealed that Dave had no drugs at all in his body—no Lithium or Luvox (fluvoxamine). He had stopped taking all medications. One should never abruptly stop taking these mood stabilizing medications or SSRI's. (Selective Serotonin Reuptake Inhibitors)

It could cause severe psychosis. The decision making part of the brain will fail to function. David was incapable of making a rational choice.

> *"Constantly aware, on your own, empty chair*
> *Versatile way, ending your sad today*
> *Pleading- you're sad today, On you're own—empty chair"*
> — *David Franchini*

No mother should ever endure such heartbreaking pain. Although at times, seeming insurmountable, as I continue to grieve, I choose to persist in living life and seeking beauty and love as David would have wanted me to.

When facing reality, I know in my heart I must choose to honor and pay tribute to my son—by living my life as happily as I can. By writing his story, presenting some of his lyrics and poetry, and offering his CD to all who care to listen, perhaps I may find some consolation.

I choose to celebrate his life and remember all the joys and fun-loving moments we shared. It gives me some peace to imagine him surrounded in a warm glowing light, free of illness, happily walking with his Dad Lino, and Our Lord.

I'm sure it is a place of indescribable color, beauty, and love. I have no fear of the day I join my David and Lino.

Note:

In one of my dreams, I asked David, "how will I know you're at peace?" He responded, "when you look at a flower, and nature; think of me."

In 2006, one year before the O.C.D. occurred, Dave bought ten, huge vases and several bags of soil. He planted a gorgeous array of flowers for me. Oh yes, I will always feel his presence and see his face when I look at them.

Ciao, Mio Dolce Figlio
See you soon my sweet son.

Riposati In Pace e Serenitá
Rest in peace and serenity.

Con Grande Amore, Mama
With the utmost love, mamma.

> *"Love is something eternal. The aspect*
> *may change, but not the essence"*
> *— Vincent Van Gogh*

DAVID

Dave's Tools of Expression And Feelings

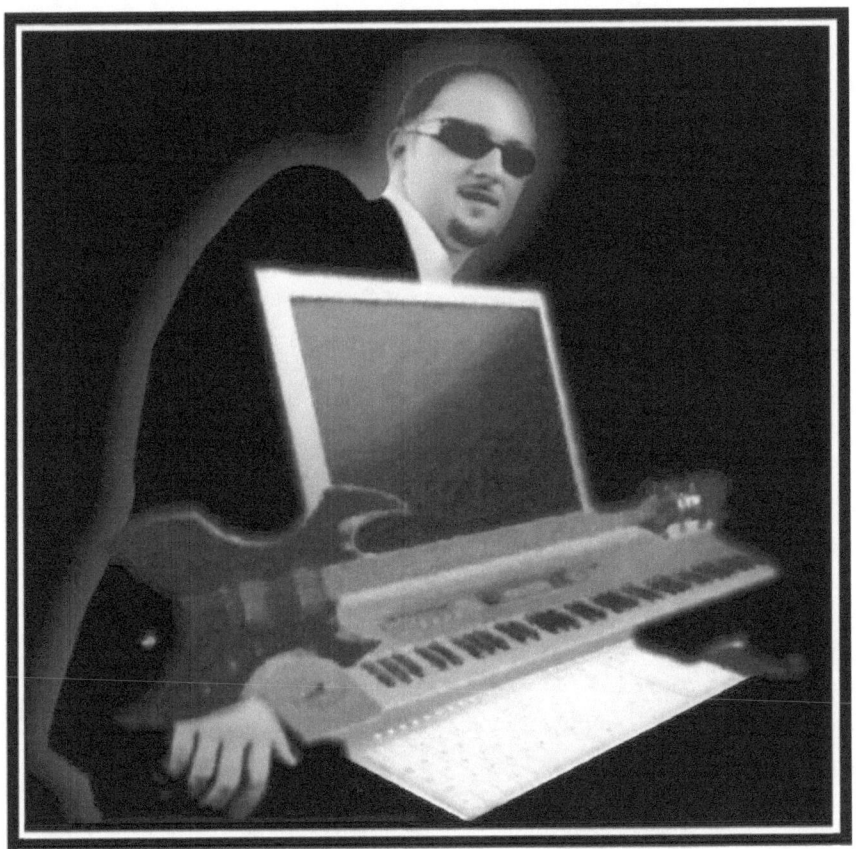

From a High Place

Coming Down From a High Place, Losing Your Grounds
Breaking Down On This Highway, Losing Your Grounds
I Wanted To Believe In It
I've Tried, Still I Try So Hard
I Wanted To Believe In It
I've Tried, Still I Try So Hard
Liquid Message Left Unspoken, Broken Essence
— by David Franchini

Part 4

David's Lyrics

*I present some of David's lyrics revealing the
despair and pain he was experiencing*

One afternoon while driving in the car with David. I said to him, "there's a part of you I'll really never know—the mysterious side; isn't that so Dave?" There was just silence—no response. Reflecting upon this, I said, "well, it's probably true for all those we love."

The complexities of our personalities can't really be fully perceived by others. The part of David that "felt", that exhibited profound emotional pain was only expressed in his lyrics. And I knew that he certainly didn't want his "mother" to read much of his writing.

It was only after he passed, that I read all his work—and it was so shockingly tragic. It felt as if it was someone else writing these painful experiences; not my son. Tragically so, I did not fully comprehend the extreme degree of his suffering.

David hid his feelings from me, his family, his friends, even the doctors and therapists. To all, his passing was utter shock and disbelief. I only know I miss him terribly, but I will make the effort to continue the healing process of this 'open wound' that remains with me to this day.

Bleed_998

Drowning in this life we live,
You're falling in too deep.
Is there a different way?
A different way to see this.

Living through our destiny,
A chance for us to see.
Hold on to memories
Still running through this time frame.

Breaking all the walls i see,
And searching endlessly.
I ask the reason why,
The meaning of our bleeding.

Chorus:
Bleeding Hands Of Mine
My Heart And Soul Are Blind
Twisted, Distorted
My Visions of Mankind.

DAVID

Broken Day

Nothing ends, forget those years
Passing by, the filthy sky clears
Back again, the rage in your eyes
Living through, emotion left aside
Digging in, damaging your pride
Take away, this emptiness inside

Loosing control – another broken day
Wonder aloud – I've got to get away

Living through emotions left aside
Digging in damaging your pride
Take away this emptiness inside

Loosing control – another broken day
Wonder aloud – I've got to get away

On your own, your plans just fall apart
You can feel, the needle in your heart
All is lost, and don't know where to start

Loosing control – another broken day
Wonder aloud – I've got to get away

DAVID

Chained

There was a time when everything went right
You look down on everything in site
I know you don't believe in anything anymore
And all the time you spent in vain here....

Push away your fears inside
Break these chains, locked deep in your mind

Everything that you know is in my head
All the words that you say have all been said
Use another excuse upon yourself
Wrapped up in lies, you're someone else

Push away your fears inside
Break these chains, locked deep in your mind

Grey line cutting through your heart
Those lies leading in-to it
Hold on something's got to change
There's time left to rearrange.

Push away your fears inside
Break these chains, locked deep in your mind

DAVID

Existence

Rise up to my grounds
Rise up to this
Shut eye and close blade
Existence won't fade

Digging in and out of your mind
Dead visions of essence
Locked deep inside your head
Dead visions of essence

Walking down these dirty streets
Million walls wide open eyes
Broken minds and broken souls
Bring you down – the hatred grows

Digging in and out of your mind
Dead visions of essence
Locked deep inside your head
Dead visions of essence

Living pain yet endlessly
Closed fist in rage ready
Your eyes, your secret lies
No more time to realize,

Digging in and out of your mind
Dead visions of essence
Locked deep inside your head
Dead visions of essence

Perfect World

Mass confusion generating lost illusion
Paranoia building up to mass hysteria
Liquid messages left unspoken, broken essence
Complicated execution vision faded

Chasing obsessions until they kill
Programmed reaction that follows your will
Facing a shift in society
Question the truth of our liberty
Pay for your justice throughout the land
Power and freedom go hand in hand

All these actions of purity
Seem so clear – yet obscure to me
As I try – to understand
How you think – and where you stand
I deny – this perfect view
A perfect world we drown into

Rearranging mental process disconnecting
Single fragment turning into deadly treatment
Tested research double-blinded system damaged

All these actions of purity
Seem so clear – yet obscure to me
How you think – and where you stand
I deny – this perfect view
A perfect world we drown into

Exit this system that shapes your path
Gather the answers that lie beneath
Government testing this human leash
Processed in line where your number's cash
Reflect the future through media control
Forced to believe in one leader for all

DAVID

Violent Movement

Around the corner of your eye
The center of your eye
The middle of your lie
Set image in the mind
Still rising but they're blind
There's only just one kind

Violent movement
Relentless this process

Building up another way
Made it easier to say
Revolution here today
Rise and fall of what we know
Watch the revolution
Watch the revolution grow

Violent movement
Relentless this process

Too Much

She's just a girl looking at me
I'm just a man staring at the world
Dancing around, standing on clouds
She held my hand, in sign of trust

Is it? - Is it too much for me?
Is it? - Is it too much for me?
Is it? - Is it too much for me?
Is it? - Is it too much for me?

Downfall

You can fall in this way
wonder how you might feel today
Senseless now and blind
leaving you behind

You can fall in this way
wonder how you might feel today
Senseless now and blind
leaving you behind

Your downfall...In process, your downfall is in my hand
your downfall...In progress, your downfall is in my hand

You can fall in this way
wonder how you might feel today
Senseless now and blind
leaving you behind

Captured Senses

Image begins to fade
Move Closer to the blade
Aggression in our eyes
Compassion in disguise

Sinful
Action
Captures
The senses
Living for today
Nothing left to say
Look deep in your soul
No grounds for control

Dig up your memories
Caught in grey velvet leaves
Releasing perfectly...
Existing Sanity

Sinful
Action
Captures
The senses
Living for today
Nothing left to say
Look deep in your soul
No grounds for control

Look deep in your soul...
No grounds for control...
Look deep in your soul

All I wanted...something senseless
All I wanted...something senseless
All I wanted...Captured senses

Untitled

Heads are down
Waiting for peace to come
No one sleeps now
That the sun is gone

Running from what you feel is wrong
What you think is right??
Falling you almost hit the ground

Sequence is moving slow
Trust your inner belief
The silence within

Her

I can see the joy in her eyes sinking in
She's locked deep down in my heart once again
Away—ten thousand miles from here
Faith was her name—Always laughing

Still with doubts and shame
Believe in yourself now
Just words I wrote for you today
She's underneath my skin once again

Church Cathedral Hall -

Jaded Sky

Laying in the rain
Living throughout constant game
Transparent obsession
Your mind is my illusion
Take away the pain
Bleeding inside leave me insane
Transparent obsession
Your mind is my illusion

Jaded face in the sky
Open up your eye, open up your eye
Jaded in the sky
Jaded.... Jaded Sky

Laying in the rain
Living throughout constant game
Transparent obsession
Your mind is my illusion
Take away the pain
Bleeding inside leave me insane
Transparent obsession
Your mind is my illusion

Jaded face in the sky
Open up your eye, open up your eye
Jaded in the sky

Divine

My own
Your own mind
This life, misbelief
Crystal...crystal leaf

Divine so in line
You're my dawn of time
Divine so in line
You're my dawn of time
Dawn of...your time

Surreal I can feel
The pain much too real
Constant reflection
Away, far away...far away...far away

Divine so in line
You're my dawn of time
Divine so in line
You're my dawn of time
Dawn of...your time

Untitled

Living pain yet endless
Closed fist in rage
Your eyes, your secret lies
No more time to realize

Losing Control

She's loosing control in her broken chair
Deep in her mind, she knows she'll get out of here
Sad image in the mind that's left alone

It's how she feels inside
No one will ever know
Maybe you'll stumble and fall
I'll be there in the black

Blistered spirit that crawls
Crystal hands that dissolve
Reach out and give me some light

Untitled

The need has taken it's own path
My thoughts collide and crash
I know your soul is in my hand
Too dark to understand

DAVID

Front Page

You're on the front page
In my home
To talk a while
About this world
Just you and me

You're on the front page
Motionless
You're on the cover of the magazine

Untitled

Descending from a cloud
I see way up in the sky
Another memory of pain
I'm reaching out from far
Much too far away
I see your face through broken glass

Untitled

Everything's secret
Look at the sky
My soul is bleeding
Question is, why?
Look at yourself now
Wondering how?

Part 5

Helpful Resources

With the world becoming smaller and smaller due to the power of the internet, I thought to myself, "what better way to reach and communicate the greatest amount of people then to create a website/blog?"

The website will be an expansion of this book. It gives me the ability to extend my arms, reach out, and take by the hand many of the untold who suffer with challenges such as these, and their families.

It allows me to continue providing new research and resources, and hopefully provide inspiration and support through any thoughts and advice I may be able to offer. I will be documenting some of my experiences with support groups, and my on-going quest for continued peace and strength .

Please feel free to visit, explore and learn more about the subject of depression and Bipolar disorder. David's CD and this book will be made available for sale on the website. All proceeds, (100%) will be donated to various organizations dedicated to the treatment and cure of mental illness.

www.davidfranchini-bipolar.blogspot.com

NATIONAL & STATE ORGANIZATIONS

National Alliance on Mental Illness (NAMI)   800-826-3632
730 N. Franklin Street, #501
Chicago, IL 60610
www.nami.org

Depression and Bipolar Support Alliance (DBSA)   800-950-6264
2107 Wilson Boulevard, #300
Arlington, VA 22201
www.dbsalliance.org

American Foundation for Suicide Prevention   800-333-2377
120 Wall Street
New York, NY 10005
www.afsp.org

National Institute of Mental Health (NIMH)   866-615-6464
6001 Executive Blvd., Rm 8184 MSC 9663   TTY: 866-415-8051
Bethesda, MD 20892
www.nimh.nih.gov

National Mental Health Consumers Self-Help Clearinghouse
1211 Chestnut Street   866-615-6464
Philadelphia, PA 19107
www.mhasp.org

DAVID

Your Rights and the
Florida Mental Health Act
(The Baker Act)

The Florida law covering both voluntary and involuntary treatment is Chapter 394 of Florida Statues - known as the Florida Mental Health Act or the Baker Act.

Florida law encourages people with mental illnesses to seek treatment voluntarily and to choose the type of treatment needed. But Florida law recognizes that some people with mental illnesses may need to be involuntarily admitted for evaluation and treatment.

The Baker Act outlines a bill of rights for the person who is mentally ill, provides a system of due process for persons receiving services in designated mental health facilities, and creates a system of community-based acute care services

A receiving facility is the central reception point for individuals who appear to need emergency mental health care. The receiving facility must ensure that persons receive needed services in the least restrictive setting and in the least intrusive manner. Consequently, receiving facilities must ensure that persons are not inappropriately admitted to community or State Hospitals.

Under the Baker Act, no one can be admitted to a State hospital without first being screened by a community mental healthy center or clinic which must certify that State hospital admission is the most appropriate placement for the individual.

Patient's Bill Of Rights

- The right to individual dignity - respect, freedom of movement, freedom from neglect or a abuse, a humane environment, privacy.

- The right to quality treatment and rehabilitation in the least restrictive setting.

- The right to receive services regardless of the ability to pay.

- The right to give, refuse, or retract express and informed consent to mental health treatment.

- The right to communicate - mail, telephone and visitors.

- The right to social relationships - exercise, recreation and social contact.

- The right to file a petition with the court questioning the cause of determination and requesting release.

- The right to participate in treatment and discharge planning.

- The right to be informed regarding patient rights and reasonable access to personal records.

- And other constitutional and legal rights, such as; confidentiality, representation, reporting grievances, voting, religious worship, work choice and compensation.

BOOK LIST

DEPRESSION OR MANIC-DEPRESSION

A Brilliant Madness .... by Patty Duke & Gloria Hochman

An Unquiet Mind .... by Kay Redfield Jamison

Darkness Visible ....by William Styron

Daughter of the Queen of Sheba .... by Jackie Lyden

Manic Depressive Illness .... by Goodwin and Jamison

Moodswings .... by Ronald Fieve, M.D.

On the Edge of Darkness .... by Kathy Cronkite

Sights Unseen...by Kaye Gibson

The Beast .... by Tracy Thompson

We Heard the Angels of Madness ....by Diane & Lisa Berger

People with Bipolar
enrich our lives.

Many famous people are believed to have been affected by bipolar disorder, based on evidence in their own writings and contemporaneous accounts by those who knew them.

It is often suggested that genius (or, at least, creative talent) and mental disorder are linked; the connection was widely publicized by Kay Redfield Jamison in Touched with Fire, although many of the diagnoses in the book are made by Jamison herself.

Ludwig van Beethoven, composer
Alastair Campbell, author
Dick Cavett, television journalist
Kurt Cobain, musician
Patricia Cornwell, American crime writer
Richard Dreyfuss, actor, BBC Documentary
Patty Duke, actress
Carrie Fisher, actress and writer
Mel Gibson, actor and director
Alexander Hamilton, politician
Linda Hamilton, actress
Kay Redfield Jamison, clinical psychologist
Rep. Patrick J. Kennedy

Margot Kidder, actress

Vivien Leigh, actress

Kristy McNichol, actress

Edvard Munch, artist.

Sir Isaac Newton, pioneering scientist and mathematician

Florence Nightingale, nurse and health campaigner

Jaco Pastorius, jazz musician

Jane Pauley, TV presenter and journalist

Jimmy Piersall, baseball player

Edgar Allan Poe, poet and writer

Emil Post, mathematician

Charley Pride, country music artist

Nina Simone, American singer

Sidney Sheldon, producer, writer

Jean-Claude Van Damme, actor

Vincent van Gogh, artist.

Kurt Vonnegut, author

FOR COMPLETE REFERENCES TO ALL OF THE ABOVE... AND MORE....
YOU CAN VISIT THE WEBSITE LISTED BELOW

http://en.wikipedia.org/wiki/List_of_people_affected_by_bipolar_disorder

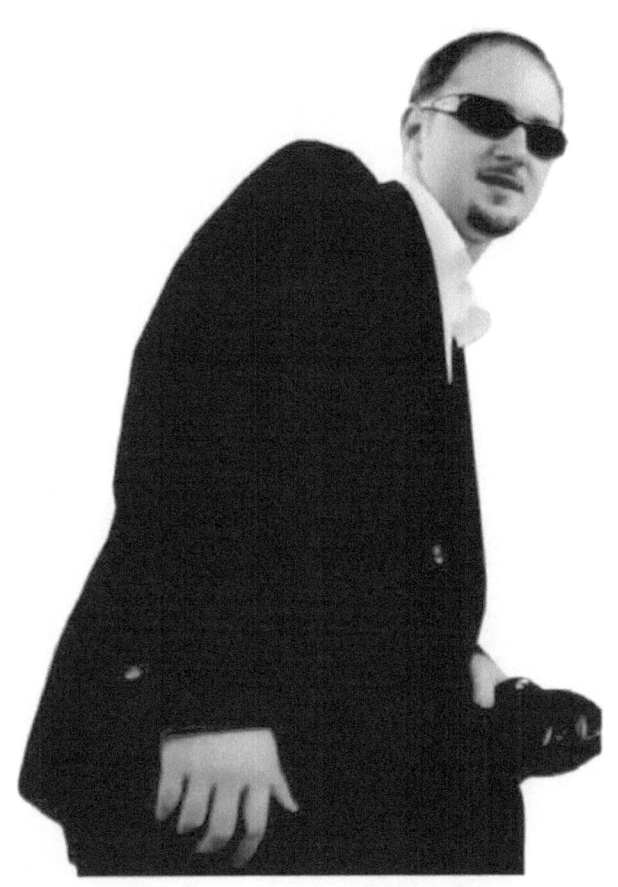

1976 — 2008

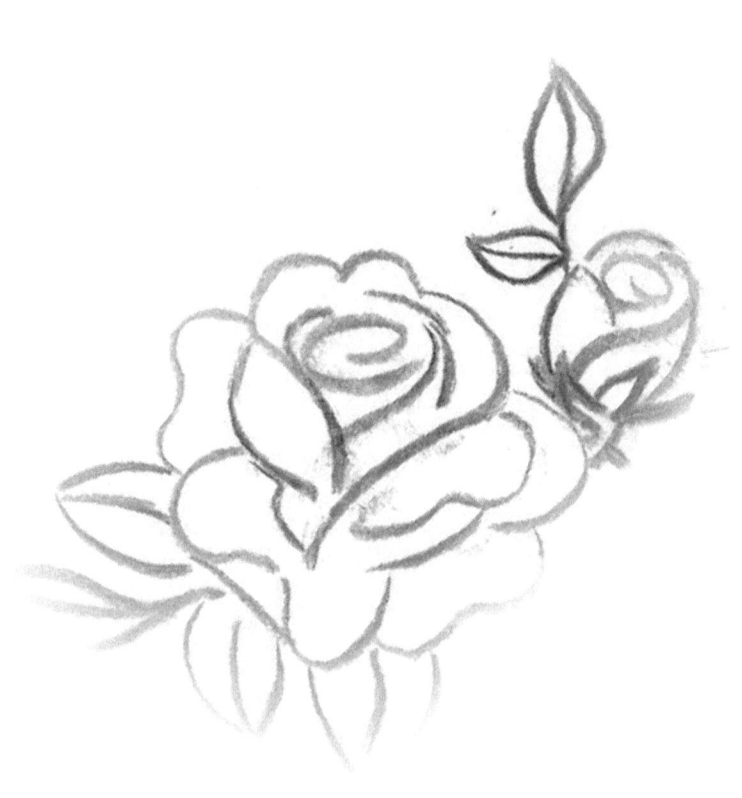

David

www.ingramcontent.com/pod-product-compliance
Lightning Source LLC
Chambersburg PA
CBHW030355290526
45785CB00004B/1756